IF YOU ARE GETTING FATTER
AND YOU DON'T KNOW WHY
It's Time to Go Back to Basics

By:
Daniel E. Ouellette

ISBN 978-1-257-91172-1

<u>Dedication</u>

*This book is dedicated to the many people
I have known throughout my life who have
been on numerous diets throughout their
lives, but just can't seem to loose their
extra weight…*

As you read this simple book of simple thoughts on the foods we eat, I want you to think about what each sentence, each paragraph, and each page really means. Don't think about what the "experts" have pushed on us for years; think about the natural process your body goes through on a daily basis.

WHY I WROTE THIS BOOK

I think about the fact that my mother's mother, Mary Hinkley, who we call Nana, turned ninety-two not that long ago. She is relatively healthy and only has a few medical issues that developed some time close to her seventieth birthday. In her late sixties she had a heart valve replaced. In her early seventies, she was diagnosed with diabetes. She regularly visited the doctor throughout her life, but this was not discovered until she was quite ill and unable to get out of bed on her own. In her eighties, she began falling. They installed a pacemaker thinking her heart would miss a beat and she would blackout. It turns out her carotid artery is partially blocked and slows the blood flow to her brain. When that happens it causes her to black out and fall. On one of those falls she broke her hip and now must walk with a walker.

I talk about my Nana for one reason. She is ninety-two and relatively healthy. Her medical issues started very late in life for her, which should be surprising considering how she ate in her younger years.

Growing up, it was not unusual for us to eat at Nana's house three, four, five or six times a week. When we did eat there, it usually was pork chops fried in real butter, meatloaf made with real eggs, pot roast floating in its own fat with potatoes and carrots soaking up that fat, ham baked in its own fatty juices, BLT's with lots of miracle whip, creamy mashed potatoes made with real butter and whole milk, home made stuffing with lots of butter, home made cookies, cakes, and brownies made with real butter or animal lard, and a whole slew of other fat-laden meals served with white bread covered with real butter. Then to top it off, most of those meals were eaten with a tall cold glass of whole milk, sometimes served with chocolate syrup mixed in for an added treat.

Then we have my father's mother, Emma Ouellette who we called Memere. She cooked old-school. Everything was filled with lard, butter, whole milk, etc… But when her children convinced her that she needed to start using those "healthy alternatives", she did. My Memere lived to be eighty-five, I believe due in part by her use of natural ingredient use as a young woman. In her late seventies my Memere had a stroke that put her in a nursing home. It wasn't caused by her use of natural products; it was caused by her use of artificial substitutes as she got older. Had she stuck with the old-school ways, I believe she would not have had a stroke.

The funny thing about all of this is that none of us were obese. Most of the family was relatively thin yet we ate foods rich in animal fats. It wasn't until diet gurus, the federal government, the processed food industry, and everyone else started telling us that butter was bad for you, switch to margarine, eggs are bad for you, switch to egg beaters, lard was bad for you, switch to vegetable oil, sugar is bad for you switch to sweet-n-low or corn syrup, whole milk is bad for you, switch to two percent or non-fat, etc…

What many people don't realize is that our bodies weren't meant to be ultra-thin. We are supposed to have a small amount of fat on them. This helps us generate heat, protect our vital organs, act as a reserve when we need a few extra calories when we exercise or participate in strenuous activities and a host of other things.

Now I am not saying that we should carry an extra one hundred pounds or even fifty pounds, but a five to ten pound fat storage won't kill you. It may even save you.

MEXICAN CO-WORKER

There was a woman I worked with a few years ago that had been born and raised in Mexico City, Mexico. We were discussing lunch plans and I mentioned going to the local buffet. She threw up her hands and said no, we couldn't go there, that place made her fat. I laughed and asked her why she said that. She explained to me that when she first moved here her new husband would take her out to eat to the buffet. There was so much food to choose from that she made a pig out of herself and got fat. Now she can't loose the weight no matter what she does. She said the only time she can loose weight is when she goes back to Mexico to visit her family.

I decided she was right, but still went to the buffet anyway. It wasn't until years later I started thinking about what she said and realized where her thinking went wrong. It wasn't because of the buffets that she had put on the weight, it was because of all the unnatural ingredients in the processed foods Americans eat.

When her mom visits the U.S., she uses our processed ingredients to cook her dishes, but when she is in Mexico, she uses natural, unprocessed foods to cook. That is why my co-worker could not loose weight unless she was visiting Mexico.

CHINESE CO-WORKER

I also worked with an older woman who was born and raised in China. She had applied for citizenship to the U.S. and eventually became a citizen. Upon moving here, she began buying her groceries at the local supermarket. She didn't know what a lot of the products were, so she stuck with what she knew how to cook.

It wasn't long when she began putting on a few extra pounds. She couldn't figure out why she was putting on the extra weight. It wasn't that she was eating anything different. She always cooked and ate at home. Her husband was also putting on the extra weight, but their diet hadn't changed at all.

It is easy to figure out what is happening here when you know what to look for. She may have been buying the same types of foods, but she was buying products that were processed using chemicals and additives that she didn't get in China.

PROCCESSED FOODS

Then we have all of those processed food companies convincing us that these substitutes are better for us and that we will be healthier by cutting down or cutting out sugars and fats. But I ask you, what has happened to the weight gain across the board since all of these "improvements" took effect?

The real reason corn syrup is used instead of sugar is the cost. It is cheaper to use corn syrup than it is to use sugar. Margarine and vegetable oil is cheaper to use than lard and real butter.

Then when you substitute margarine for real butter in the processing of foods, you need to add more artificial flavorings to make the stuff taste good. Key word here is: ARTIFICIAL.

Some people are going to say that people are living longer because of the changes in their diets. FALSE. People are living longer because of the changes in other habits such as quitting smoking, visiting the doctor more often and getting treatment for common illnesses that use to kill people when left untreated, etc... It has nothing to do with switching from high fat foods.

Again, look at the waistline of many Americans. It has steadily grown over the years since switching to these food substitutes, artificial ingredients, and other non-healthy alternatives.

I'm not going to quote any experts because it seems the experts are the ones who have convinced us that natural foods are bad for us.

I have a challenge for each of you. Go through your kitchen and throw out your margarine, vegetable oil, low-fat or fat-free milk, sugar substitutes, egg substitutes

Places like McDonald's use to be a great place to eat. It was our special treat as kids. That was when they used lard and not some oil substitute. When the general public pushed them into using "healthier alternatives" they loved the idea because it was cheaper. What resulted from the change was more unhealthy Americans getting fatter and having more health issues. So now the public condemns McDonald's for its unhealthy menu and insists they offer healthier alternatives such as apple slices and other such things. What McDonald's needs to do is return to its roots and switch back to lard.

The number of strokes and heart attacks has increased considerably over the years. Have you ever wondered why? Have you ever stopped to wonder what has changed to allow this to happen? With all of the advances in medicine, why have they increased?

Have you ever noticed that the price of "diet food" is higher than the full fat alternatives? I mentioned earlier it was cheaper to manufacture foods with the alternative ingredients, so why does diet food cost us more? Because the manufacturers have us believing that diet food is better for you so it should cost more. The reality is, it costs them less to make and they charge us more, so their overall profits are much greater. That is a great incentive to making sure the general public continue to purchase and consume these types of product so they can continue to rake in the high profits for their companies.

Do you know what the side effects of eating foods made with "healthy alternative" ingredients are? Hunger, cravings, over-eating, a thought process that says we can have more because it is "diet" food. Do you know what side effect "diet" food doesn't have on you? Weight-loss. Some people may actually loose weight while on a diet, but that is because they are thinking about the amount of food they are eating and trying not to over-indulge. Some are actually exercising more too. That is where the weight-loss is coming from, not the "diet" food. The diet food is actually hampering your weight loss.

Try this instead. Get rid of all of the "diet" foods in your house. Bring back the natural products that the "experts" told you to get rid of. Cook your own meals using those real foods and follow a plan as though you are on a diet. Cut down on your food intake and get up off that sofa and walk around a bit. You will see the weight start to go away when you are not feeding your body all of those unhealthy "healthy substitutes".

Here is what happens in your body when you cook with vegetable oil, margarine, low-fat mayo/miracle whip, etc: Your body looks at that substance and wonders what it is. Since it doesn't know what it is it stores it as fat so it can digest it later. Your body never figures out what it is, so it leaves it where it is.

Lard on the other hand, goes into your body. Your body immediately recognizes it as natural animal fat and processes it out of your body. Case closed, body fat avoided.

The same goes with corn syrup. It is so over-processed that your body does not recognize it. So again, it stores it as fat. Sugar is a common, natural substance. Your body knows what to do with it. It takes what it needs and sends it on through the system.

So what is the deal with eggs? According to the experts today are they good for you or bad for you? What about potatoes. They are supposed to contain enough calories to equal a cup of sugar. Wake up people... Potatoes contain NATURAL calories. No artificial sweeteners in there. The food industry can't make a lot of money off a baked potato, but it certainly can off imitation potato flakes. Read the package of a box of dried potato flakes. It may say made with real potatoes, but how processed do you want your food to be? And what chemicals did they add to those potatoes? Are they "fortified" with artificial vitamins and minerals? That is because there is nothing nutritious about dried potato flakes without the "sprayed-on" chemical nutrients. Your body can process the natural ingredients in a potato, but has no idea what to do with the processed potato flakes from a box...

EAT WHAT YOU CRAVE

Have you ever been around a dog that eats grass? Do you know why that dog is eating the grass? The dog knows that their body needs something and eats it. A dog eats because it is hungry. A dog drinks because it is thirsty. A dog begs for treats because we humans have taught them to beg for it.

Most Americans no longer eat to live, they live to eat. That needs to change. But we are not going to be able to change that until we get rid of the over-processed, unnatural foods that we stuff our faces with daily. Processed, unnatural foods are the reason we are over-weight and obese. The cravings artificial sweeteners and unnatural products produce cause us to over-eat every day. If we switched back to an all-natural diet, we would quickly loose the weight.

Once you switch back, start to listen to your body's cravings. If it is craving a baked potato, eat it. If it is craving a brownie, eat it. If it is craving a glass of ice-cold milk, drink it.

When you switch back, your body will most likely "freak out". For most of your life it has been trying to process all of those unnatural ingredients you have been force-feeding it. When you switch back your body is going to wonder what is happening. The first thing that may happen is a slight increase in your weight. Be patient during this process, it will eventually turn itself around.

The second thing that happens is your cravings start to decrease. There are two types of cravings. One is the psychological cravings. You are used to eating certain things at certain times, so your mind is telling you to eat. Those are the cravings you need to ignore. The second type of craving is the one that you need to listen to. It is the cravings your body is sending you. Your body knows when it needs something and will tell you what it is in the form of a craving. Distinguishing between the two is the hard part, but it is something you yourself need to determine. Give it plenty of time and don't give up.

One of the other important things to follow is to not skip a meal. If your body is having a craving, give in and feed it. If not, you throw off your system's natural balance. Just like when your vehicle needs gas, you pull into the gas station and fill it, so does your body need fuel.

ALL NATURAL

When it contains the words "all natural" they are referring to the initial ingredients. What they are not telling you is that the "all natural" part of it is lost during the processing of the product. Corn syrup is all natural when it starts out, but over-processing it for use creates an unnatural substance.

Take cold cereal for instance. Cold cereal might start out with natural ingredients, but it is processed, pressed, squeezed, cooked, dried, manipulated into looking like flakes and berries and then coated with vitamins and minerals to meet federal standards. The only way these cereals can claim to meet federal guidelines is by adding natural and artificial ingredients to the outside of the cereal by spraying it on. You would be better off eating bacon, eggs and toast with a glass of whole milk. But be sure to fry the eggs using a little bit of lard and smear the toast with a little bit of real butter.

Not only will you be satisfied, you will not be craving a mid-morning snack of potato chips or one of those "healthy" snack bars everyone seems to eat in-between meals.

Your mind won't be telling you to eat these because your body is not filled with artificial ingredients and chemicals, And it is not lacking the natural foods it needs to survive.

If you eat a healthy breakfast as mentioned above, by the time lunch rolls around, you will be hungry again because your body has processed the natural ingredients you gave it for breakfast. So be sure to feed your body again with a meal filled with natural ingredients and don't opt for a microwave meal or overly-processed fast food lunch!

GETTING BACK TO BASICS

Take this book with you to your kitchen. Open up the refrigerator/freezer and remove the following:

- artificially sweetened juices
- non-whole milk
- low fat dressings
- imitation whipped cream
- low fat ice cream
- popsicles

- margarine
- cheese made w/o whole milk
- diet sodas
- egg substitutes
- frozen dinners

Now open your cupboards and pull everything out that you can eat. If an item contains any of the following ingredients, throw them out:

- Corn syrup
- fructose
- nutra-sweet
- trans-fat
- saccharine

- artificial sweetener
- sweet-n-low
- equal
- polyunsaturated fat

or any words you can't pronounce. If the word sounds like a chemical, chances are great that it is. You don't need chemicals in your food!

Anything containing the following words on the front of the package also need to be thrown in the garbage:

- low-fat
- diet
- sugar free
- healthy
- all natural

- fat-free
- low sugar
- low sodium
- healthier

Use caution when disposing of these unwanted foods. They could be hazardous to your pets if they get into them...

I'm also wondering if it is safe to dispose of them in the landfill. The chemicals might leach into our ground water...

Now that you have taken the bad foods out, start filling your pantry with the good stuff. Those would include the following:

- real butter
- whole milk
- regular salad dressing
- real potatoes
- beef
- chicken w/skin
- bacon
- pasta

- animal lard
- real cheese
- eggs
- regular ice cream
- pork
- sugar
- breads

The list goes on. When enough Americans wake up and realize what the food industry is doing to us, they will begin shopping like they should and these large corporations will have no choice but to change their ways and stop killing us slowly.

THE REASON I CHANGED MY EATING HABITS

The day before my fortieth birthday I had a heart attack caused by a blocked artery leading back into my heart. Luckily I had the foresight to go to the emergency room when I did. Within minutes of entering the emergency room, I had a full-blown heart attack. The cardiologist who operated and put the stent in my heart told me I was a very lucky man. Had I not been in the ER at the time of my attack, I would have been dead. There would not have been enough time to get me the help I needed.

That night the hospital staff drew blood and ran tests. My cholesterol level was two hundred and ten, which the doctor said was not very high. My blood pressure was one thirty over eighty, which the doctor said was elevated, but not high. He said they prescribe blood pressure lowering medication after your blood pressure reaches one forty or more over ninety or more.

When I discussed my cholesterol with the cardiologist, he explained that he does not put much merit in cholesterol levels. He said there were two different types of strokes and this is the best way for me to explain it:

Type number one: Once having a type number one stroke, your chances of recovering are quite low. These types of strokes are debilitating and when they occur, there is significant damage to the surrounding brain tissue. People with low cholesterol tend to have these types of strokes.

Type number two: Once you have a type number two stroke, your chances of recovery are very high. There is typically very little damage to the brain tissue. People who have these types of strokes typically have high cholesterol.

So the next time you pop that cholesterol lowering synthetic drug, ask yourself which type of stroke you want to have and also ask yourself what unnatural chemical you just popped into your body.

Personally, I would rather have stroke that I can recover from and not worry about the added chemicals I am taking.

So with this information in hand, I started looking at what I was putting into my body every day. Reading the ingredients labels of the food I was eating almost caused me another heart attack. So I slowly began getting rid of the processed foods starting with margarine, vegetable oil, low fat milk, and such. I then started working on the commercially created snacks that I ate. The reason why an old-fashioned home made cake tastes so good is because of the lack of chemicals and artificial flavorings it contains.

It didn't stop there. I started buying beef, chicken, and pork products to make my own foods and slowed down on eating prepackaged, over-processed foods containing processed meat byproducts.

Guess what happened! I started feeling better. I started craving less and less junk food like potato chips, snack cakes, cookies, etc... I did develop a few cravings though, but those craving were for good foods like mashed potatoes, green beans, cucumbers, and such. I got those cravings because my body started telling what it needed...

So all-in-all it is up to you to decide. You decide if you want to continue to kill yourself with all of those chemicals, food additives, over-processed food replacements, and whatever else the "experts" tell you are bad for you.

HEARTBURN

Do you suffer from heartburn or acid reflux? Do you drink a lot of reverse osmosis water throughout the day? Do you use ice in your drink that was processed through reverse osmosis? Chances are they are related. While you may be blaming the heartburn and acid reflux on the soda, it really is the ice processed through reverse osmosis that is causing it. Most restaurants and convenience stores use this type of filtering for their water and ice, so stop blaming it on the food and drink and start blaming it on the filtration system.

It is also most likely that any beverage that has been bottled or canned has had the water content filtered through reverse osmosis.

So why hasn't anyone been able to connect the rise in heartburn and acid reflux to the process in which we manufacture our beverages? Because someone with money will loose money if the truth gets out.

One thing that I mentioned before is, why do we continue to take medications for symptoms but we never try to figure out the cause? Heartburn has a cause, so why are doctors not trying to figure out what that is? Because it is easier to prescribe medications to take care of the symptoms than it is to admit that our food and beverage additives are causing it. It isn't the foods themselves, it is the processes and the additives.

24

MEDICATIONS

Do you take a lot of different medications and you are having trouble sleeping, or have trouble loosing weight, or having trouble going to the bathroom regularly? Take a look at your medication. Every medication produced today has side effects. Some of those side effects are deadly. And they are even worse when mixed with other medications. The majority of medications out there are synthetic, man-made, chemicals. How does your body react to unnatural substances?

Now I am not advocating that you stop taking your medication. That is something you need to decide with help from your doctor. But remember, doctors are given "incentives" for prescribing certain medications, and while no doctor will ever admit it, they do.

Find a new doctor. Find a doctor that is willing to work with you to develop a more natural method for controlling your illness. Medications are not a long-term solution, they are a method to alleviate temporary symptoms until the root cause of the illness can be determined and fixed.

Take high blood pressure for example. Most doctors put you on medication to lower it instead of telling you the truth. The truth being you need to loose weight. You need to exercise more. You need to stop filling your body with unhealthy processed foods. You need to stop stressing over the little things in life.

Back when my great grandparents were alive, they lived in the country on a dairy farm. They ate real butter that they made. They ate real ice cream that they made. They drank real whole milk from their own cows. They baked cakes and other stuff using real buttermilk. They ate yard eggs from the chickens they raised on corn. They butchered chickens, pigs, and cows for the meat they ate. They cooked that meat in lard. They cooked bacon and sausage from the pigs they slaughtered. They didn't have corn syrup, margarine, vegetable oil and processed foods. Yet they both lived into their late seventies and eighties and they didn't take cholesterol lowering drugs or blood pressure drugs. They most likely didn't even have preventive vaccines growing up either.

Today's commercial cows, chickens, and pigs are raised on by-products and not their natural diet of grass and grains. Its no wonder why commercially raised animals need to be injected with hormone and anti-biotic chemicals that end up in the meats and dairy products we consume.

ADDITIONAL POINTS

Your body contains salt. If you have ever tasted your own tears then you know that. So why do doctors and nutritionists warn you about eating too much salt.

Because table salt is iodized and that process is what makes salt bad for you. If you like salt then switch to all-natural sea salt that is not iodized. You don't need as much to flavor your food and it is much healthier for you. Better yet, get rid of the table salt anyway, then you won't be tempted to use it on anything.

Tylenol, Motrin, and other similar pain relievers are not good for you. First off they are chemicals. Second, they lower your body temperature. When you lower your body temperature you lower your body's ability to burn calories. So when you over use these pain relievers you will put on weight because your body doesn't need the calories you just ate to keep the fire burning. And what happens to calories when they don't get used? They are stored as fat for later use.

What about the rise in the number of people being diagnosed with diabetes? Every year it seems as though there are more people being diagnosed with diabetes and the age is getting lower. Look at the processed food additives as the culprit.

My grandmother use to use a lot of molasses and brown sugar to cook. I noticed she doesn't any more. Now she uses caro syrup and white sugar. Read the bottles of both and you will see for yourself which ones are the all natural products.

GOOD GENES

There have been quite a few times when I hear people comment that I come from a very long line of ancestors with good genes. Growing up, I hade the privilege of knowing my great-grandparents on my mother's side. I knew my mother's mother (who is ninety-two) this year, my mother's father who was close to ninety, if not in his nineties, when he died, and my father's mother who was eighty-five when she passed. I have also known a large number of great aunts and great uncles well into their seventies, eighties, and nineties.

Good genes had nothing to do with it. It was the good old-fashioned eating habits that made it happen. Plus the fact that none of them stopped long enough to stress about what they ate. They were either busy running a farm or working hard in a textile mill and eating what they grew up eating. They got their exercise daily by not sitting at an office desk typing on the computer, or sitting at home on the sofa watching television. When they weren't working they were still moving around at either a dance, or family gathering, or swimming to cool off. And when they weren't doing either of those, they were in bed getting their rest.

I was lucky enough to have grown up in this wonderful family. They taught me how to eat right, but as the years went by and "experts" got involved, we all started moving away from the healthy way to eat and started filling our freezers, refrigerators, cupboards, and bodies with over-processed, unnatural, chemically altered foods. That is when the health issues started appearing. It wasn't a breakdown in our good genes, it was a breakdown in the way we live and eat.

So I ask you this. With a family who has absolutely no heart attack history going back four generations, how is it that I was lucky enough to have a heart attack at the age of thirty-nine and was able to come to the realization that I was killing my body with things our experts call nutritious foods? Go back to the basics and teach your children those same basics. Maybe not in my lifetime, but maybe in the generations to follow, they will see where the experts went wrong and be able to reverse the damage they have caused the entire population.

HOW TO DO IT

You are now close to the end of the book and you are beginning to think about some of the major points this book makes. You are asking yourself if this stuff is true. Without hesitation, I can tell you that yes it is true.

So now you want to know what you can do to make changes in your life. I suggest you start by emptying out your kitchen as I mentioned earlier in this book.

Then start planning meals that avoid processed foods. If you don't like to cook, find someone that does.

Find an old cookbook that is easy to follow and has simple recipes. Dig out your mother's or grandmother's recipe book or cards and start there. Be sure not to use imitation and chemically altered ingredients.

Buy a crockpot, or dig yours out of the bottom cabinet. Clean it up and set it on the counter. Your crockpot could be your best friend. Foods that are slow-cooked usually taste the best. The natural flavors have time to blend together forming a mouth-watering experience so delicious you can't imagine ever going back to your old ways.

One of my favorite meals is pot roast, potatoes, and carrots. My family recipe for pot roast is simple and delicious.

You can't go wrong if you follow these simple steps. I like to make mine at night and refrigerate the entire crockpot dish in the refrigerator. Then in the morning I take it out and pop it into the crockpot base and cook it all day.

Pot Roast

1. Heat up your frying pan to medium high.
2. Throw in a half a stick of butter
3. Put the roast in the pan and turn over until all sides are seared.
4. Turn down the frying pan and put the roast into the crockpot.
5. Add 2 cups of hot water and a large chopped onion to the frying pan and simmer 15-20 minutes.
6. Peal and cube potatoes and toss into the crockpot.
7. Peal and slice carrots and put into crockpot.
8. Chop up 2-3 stalks of celery and add to crockpot.
9. Pour the frying pan contents into the crockpot.
10. Simmer all day on low.

You know have a meal made with all-natural ingredients that you can be proud to serve to your family.

This same recipe can be made in an electric roasting pan set on low, but be sure to place everything into a roasting bag so that it doesn't dry out.

It really only takes a little thought and planning to feed your family the right meals. Once you get the hang of it, you will be cooking like the pros.

Think about the cooking shows on television. You don't see them cooking with over-processed foods. Most of the good cooks use butter and natural sea salt. They use natural ingredients and that is why their food tastes so good.

SEVEN YEARS LATER

I will be celebrating my seventh year since my heart attack and my seventh year of restructuring my life and my seventh year of changing the way I eat, and I must say, that I am feeling the healthiest I have felt in many years. Of course I am getting older, so I may be a bit slower, but I can feel the difference these changes have made in my life.

I no longer worry about what my cholesterol level is, I no longer worry about what my blood pressure is. I no longer ignore the cravings my body sends me. And again, I feel the best I have felt in years.

Since my heart attack and diet change I have not had a migraine. I use to suffer through them a few times a year, every year since I was about fourteen. In the past seven years, I haven't had one migraine. I used to have multiple headaches every week. Now I have one or two a year. It doesn't take an expert to determine what has changed to relive the cause of my headaches and migraines? I attribute it to the limiting of unnatural ingredients I eat every day.

So called "Experts" and other people will come up with a whole boatload of reasons why this type of diet is wrong. They will list numerous research trials to try to disclaim this book, but all I can say is that I know what works for me and I know it will work for you.

I don't think I need to remind you, but I will anyway...

Moderation is the key ingredient with any food you put into your body, so use a little common sense while enjoying your all-natural, chemical-free, unprocessed, delicious meal!

MY DISCLAIMER

- I am not a medical doctor, nor have I attended classes to become a doctor.
- I am not a nutritionist and have not attended classes to become one.
- I do not work for a pharmaceutical company, nor have I ever worked for one.
- I am not an agriculturist, I have never had training to become one, nor have I worked for one.
- I am not a chemist, I have never had a chemistry class, and I have never worked for one.
- I am not a professional cook, I have never had training to be a professional cook, but I have worked at a grill years ago.
- I do not now nor have I ever worked for a federal government agency that regulates or oversees anything related to food, drugs, or animal products.
- I love to cook for myself and others, and I love to eat rich healthy foods prepared at home.

So, with the above information in hand, it is easy to see that I have not been swayed by the misconceptions forced upon us by these entities, and am therefore qualified to render a purely reasonable conclusion to the fact that we as Americans are doing ourselves harm by allowing the above mentioned entities the ability to force-feed misinformation to us daily.

At no time have I ever referenced any study, research, paper, or trial conducted by any of the above mentioned entities to reach any conclusion contained in this book, nor have I referenced any material other than my family's recipes that used all-natural ingredients to prepare.

I am now in the process of converting my family's recipes back to their original ingredients.

www.ingramcontent.com/pod-product-compliance
Lightning Source LLC
Chambersburg PA
CBHW061233280526
45784CB00006B/2744